I0711683

a Magnificent Body with Intermittent Fasting

5 Easy Steps

Dr. Marijke Verkerk

www.drmarijkeverkerk.com

CONTENTS

The key to a Magnificent Body

This book provides you with the most relevant information, and proven tips. These are all of the key basics you need to know in order to make an informed decision about whether Intermittent Fasting is for you. The five easy steps discussed here will help you jump-start your intermittent fasting plan and quickly integrate it into your lifestyle. Find valuable tips and recommendations to help your fasting routine go more smoothly– and help you get the most out of intermittent fasting.

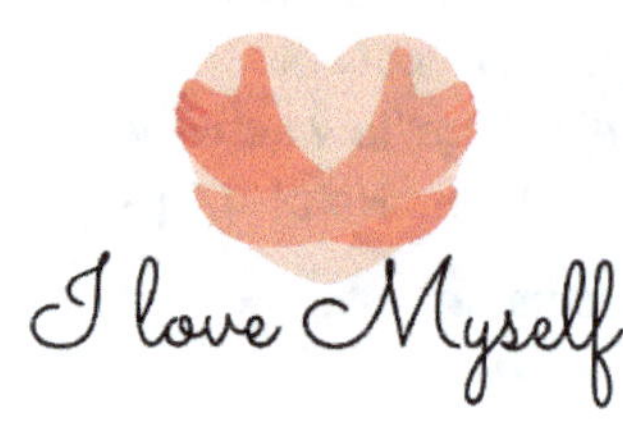

I love Myself

BODY | MIND | SPIRIT

Inside you, there is an intelligence that is always working in your favor wanting to heal your body. When we eat, this intelligence needs to put its priorities to digesting food and when we are continually eating 5 to 6 meals, including snacks, this intelligence is always working on the immediate situation, which is digesting food. And when we take food out of the equation, a whole chemical reaction is going to occur in your body.

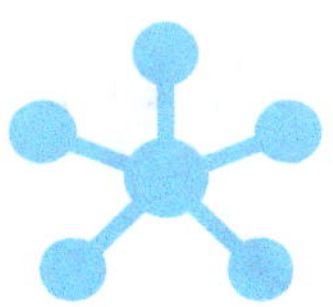

Why Intermittent Fasting?

The main reason is that it's not a traditional diet. Whether your goal is to lose weight or simply boost your overall health and vitality, intermittent fasting does not restrict you to specific foods or involve calorie-counting. You simply abstain from eating during fasting hours and eat what you want during eating hours – within reason, of course!

It's this flexibility that makes intermittent fasting so popular and very easy to adopt as a lasting lifestyle habit.

CHAPTER 1:

What is Intermittent Fasting?

Intermittent fasting is a way of eating based on periods of mini-fasts.

Most people eat 5-6 small meals a day, with intermittent fasting, you have either one meal a day with a window of 24 hours of fasting until the next meal the next day.

Or two meals a day with a fasting window of 20 hours and an eating window of 3-4 hours between meals.

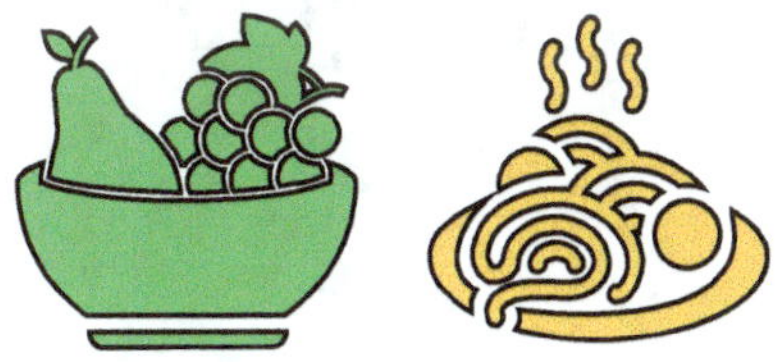

Is Intermittent Fasting a Hype?

Absolutely not! Intermittent Fasting has become a lifestyle choice for millions of people, with many more coming on board.

As research continues to discover and confirm its seemingly endless benefits.

Fasting has been practiced for centuries by various cultures worldwide for both health and spiritual benefits. It is only recently that it has become known in the West as a healthy lifestyle choice.

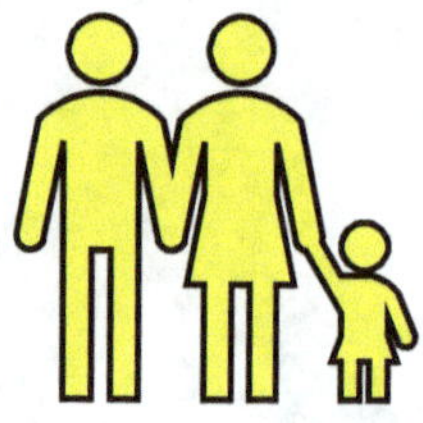

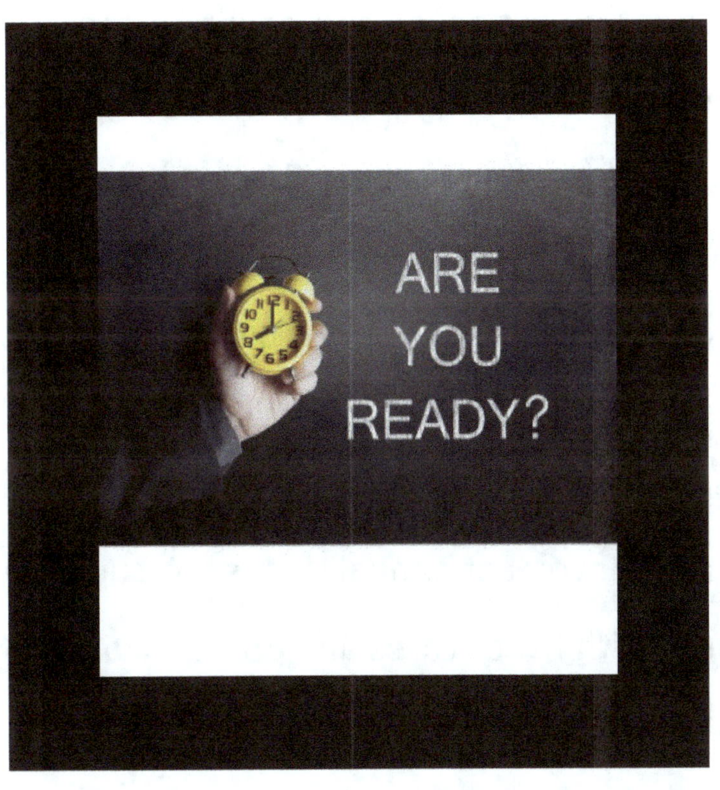
ARE
YOU
READY?

Let Your Body Do the Work

When you eat a high carbohydrate or a high protein meal the body gets a high spike of insulin. Insulin will help the body turn blood sugar (glucose) into energy. Your body stores it in your muscles, fat cells, and liver to use later when your body needs it, that takes about 8 to 10 hours. If you eat a meal that is low sugared with fewer carbs and protein, your insulin level will not be as high, and glucose will start coming down a lot quicker. But intermittent fasting begins at the moment when you stop eating.

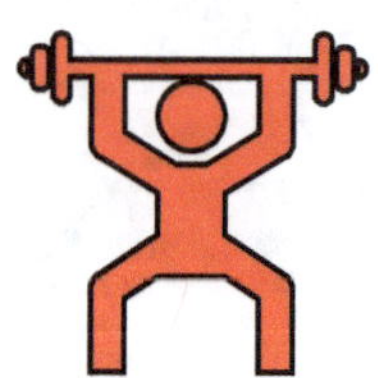

CHAPTER 2: The Growth Hormone

To speed up all the chemical reactions that the body will have from fasting the intake of carbs and protein has to be very low. Around 12 hours of not eating from your last meal the Growth-hormone will kick in. Growth hormone plays an essential factor in the ageing process, as after the age of 30, the body stops making it. Growth hormone also called the fitness hormone, and the fountain of youth is the bodies primary fat-burning hormone that builds muscle, slows down the ageing process improves memory focus and concentration.

The Fountain of Youth

Our body is full of protein found in our muscles skin and hair, nails tendons and ligaments. Growth hormone regenerates and preserves protein in the body. Children have lots of growth hormones, but in time our body produces less of it. But when you start doing fasting regularly, your growth hormone is going to kick in around that 12 hour of not eating, again. Research is showing that the growth hormone increases with 1300 percent just from 12 to 13 hours of fasting. A good reason to love the intermittent fasting lifestyle.

Ketones

What happens after 13 hours is that your body is starting to sense that no more food is coming. The body is going to make a shift from working to burn sugar, to working to burn fat. This is called ketones production, which is especially important for those of you who want to lose weight. The more ketones a body produces the more healing will occur in the cells of your body and your brain.

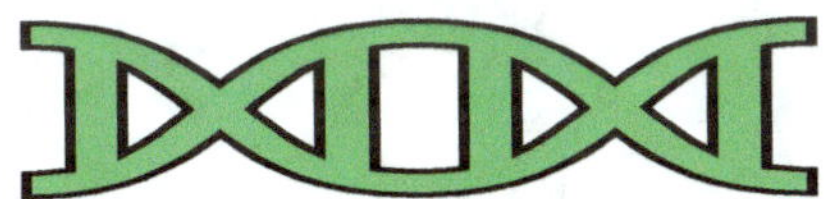

Autophagy

At 17 hours autophagy is kicking in, autophagy is when the cells realize that the blood sugar levels are going down and there is no more food coming in, and they start looking for food within the cells and they eat the toxins within the cells and start to detoxify itself. So, at 17 hours, both autophagy and the growth hormone, are switched on.

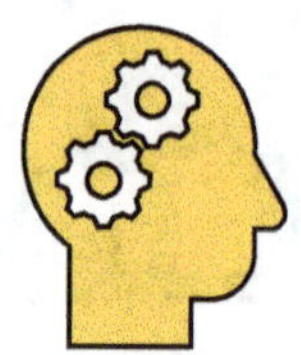

Happy Hormones

When you extend the fast up to 24 hours, three major organs are starting to repair, your intestinal stem cells are starting to regenerate, and your body starts to create more fertilizing proteins for the brain. So, you're getting intestinal repair, ketones, autophagy, and your neurons in the brain are getting repaired.
When the neuron levels in the brain go up the serotonin level goes up as well. Serotonin is a hormone that makes you feel happy.

Does fasting change your genes?

Research also shows that from 24 hours up the blood pressure and inflammation go down. There's healing in the digestive system because it finally has the chance to relax. Fasting is a potent trigger for turning off or turning on your genes.

A gene is a blueprint or code for building proteins that play an essential role in the body from making hormones to releasing stored glucose for fuel. When you fast, the cholesterol gene becomes more sen-sitive, and the number of receptors in-creases.

Source: National Library of Medicine

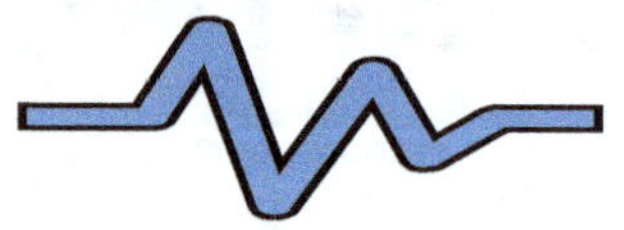

I.F benefits

Weight loss is the most common reason for people to try intermittent fasting. Researchers are discovering that when we eat may be just as important as what we eat. We learned about Autophagy, the body's ability to recycle unhealthy toxins, that supports the immune system, especially in your bone tissue and drops inflammation. Intermittent fasting also helps the cells to resist stress and build an anti-oxidant network. So, let's list the benefits of intermittent fasting and see how it goes beyond weight loss:

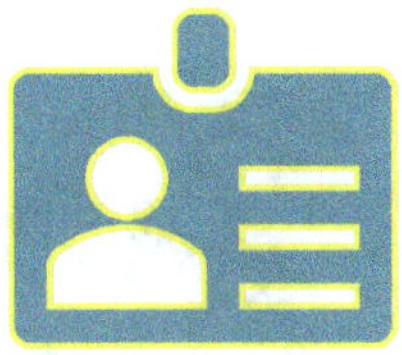

Various Health FAQ's

- I.F Increases Fertilizing proteins for the brain.

- I.F Promotes Regeneration of Stem cells.

- I.F improves metabolism / weight loss

- I.F improves muscular development.

- I.F improves your immune system and overall health.

- I.F improves your Skin quality / Fountain of youth.

- I.F improves mental functions.

- I.F Increases the Happy Hormones.

- I.F Promotes Growth Hormone.

- I.F Stimulates Autophagy.

- I.F helps Build an anti-oxidant network.

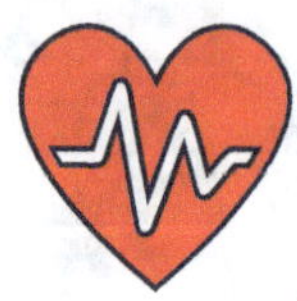

Who Intermittent Fasting Is Not For?

Intermittent fasting is not for everyone. There are certain conditions where intermittent fasting can be harmful to health. You absolutely must not fast, or at the very least consult a doctor if:

- You are pregnant.
- You are breastfeeding.
- You are anemic.
- You have a history of eating disorders.
- You have diabetes.
- You have a heart condition.
- You are under 18.
- You are on medications that must be taken during meals.

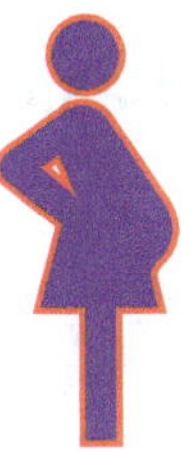

CHAPTER 3:

The Five Simple Steps

The benefits of intermittent fasting can immensely improve your quality of life. Before proceeding further although intermittent fasting is risk-free it is advisable to check with your doctor first.

So, are you ready to quick-start your intermittent fasting program? Intermittent fasting needs no complicated preparations and it is practically cost-free (unless you choose to invest in supplements or special foods). All you need to do is quick-start your intermittent fasting routine with these five basic steps.

STEP 1: Define your Goal

If your primary goal is to lose those extra pounds, you will have to watch the amount you eat more carefully than someone who's not looking to lose weight. You need not necessarily restrict calories, but consume less calorie-rich foods, avoid sugar and snacking between meals and perhaps cut out deserts. This will optimize your fasting and help you reach your weight loss goal much faster. You may also consider adding a workout routine on non-fast days to tone your body as the pounds come off.

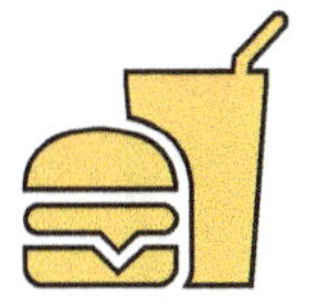
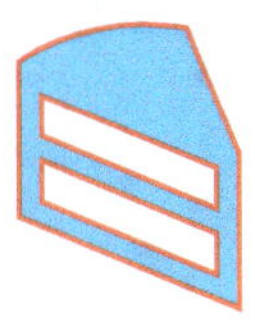

BRAIN FOODS

Some people fast to improve their mental strength such as memory and concentration. In this case, you would want to eat more brain foods that help stimulate your mental focus and cognitive function.

Some Foods that stimulate the brain are:

- Coffee
- Fatty fish
- Blueberries
- Turmeric
- Broccoli
- Pumpkin seeds
- Dark chocolate
- Nuts
- Green tea
- Eggs

Overall Health and Wellbeing

Some people fast simply to reap all the benefits and to feel healthier and more energized. Fasting, in general, is a great detoxifier of the body and just leaves you looking better and feeling better. Some of the first benefits you will notice is improved complexion, healthier hair and nails. You feel calmer, and your digestion will be more balanced.

In this case, you can be more flexible with what you eat as long as you are focusing on good nutrition.

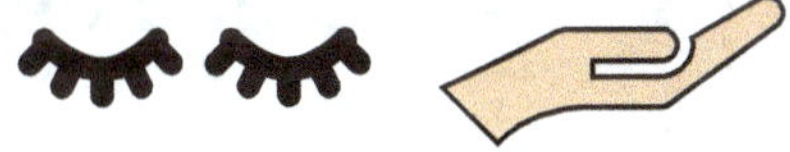

For glowing, toned and clear skin

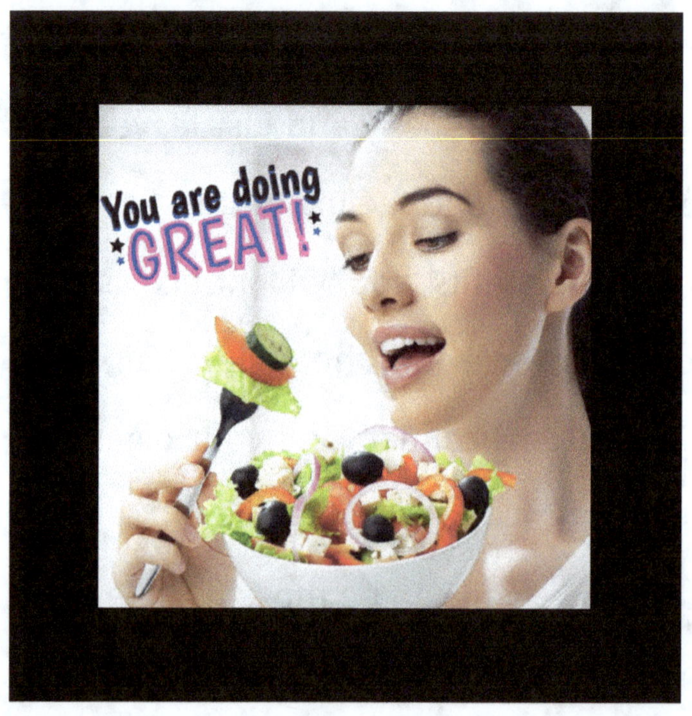

Eat well, sleep well and exercise

STEP 2: Choose A Fasting Plan

There are different intermittent fasting plans and variations of them, but the following three are the most popular and most commonly practiced:

- **The 16/8 method**

With this plan you fast for a full 16 hours with an eating window of 8 hours every day. I would recommend that you start your fast after dinner, around 7 or 8 pm. Then break your fast the next day around noon. You will likely feel less hungry after a good diner, while the other 7 or 8 hours will be taken up by sleep. After breaking your fast by noon, the next day will feel like you are having a late breakfast.

You can enjoy a light meal or snack in the end of the afternoon, ending your fasting day with a delicious and nutritious dinner.

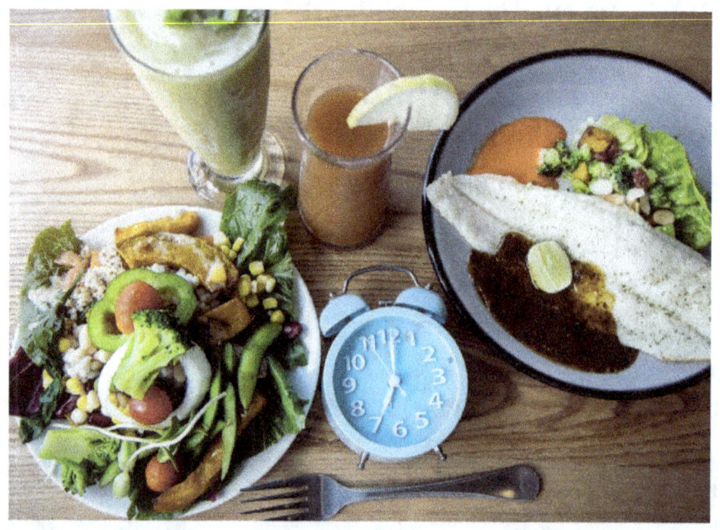

I recommended that you practice this method by alternating two fasting days with two days where you eat normally. More experienced fasters sometimes alternate three fasting days with three normal eating days.

Keep Your Body Hydrated

Fluids like water, unsweetened coffee, tea or herbal tea are allowed during fasting hours and in fact, are highly recommended to keep your body hydrated. This plan may seem overwhelming; however, if you choose it, try to start with a shorter fasting window of 10 or 12 hours and bit by bit build-up to the total 16 hours. You can also consider playing around with the times that suit your lifestyle best. For example, if you are an early riser, you can plan to break your fast at 10 am. In this case, you're eating window would be until 6 pm. Play with it and find the hours you are most comfortable with.

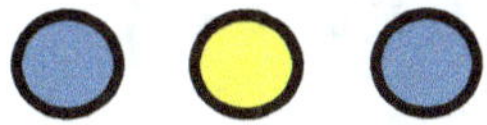

- **The 5:2 plan**

This method is easy to explain.

You eat like you usually do for five days, and the remaining two days reduce your calorie intake to a quarter which is about 600 – 800 calories.

 You divide the 600 – 800 calories over three meals on the two fasting days. This way will drastically cut the calories and lose weight. The only challenge with this plan is dividing the low-calorie intake over your meals. Some fasters cut out carbs and fruits and fill up on protein and nuts. This plan leaves enough space and a bit of creativity to eat pretty well on these two days.

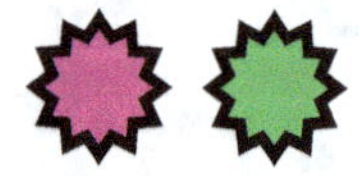

- **24-hours Fast**

The 24 hours fast is known as the eat-stop-eat plan for one or two days a week. So, if you start fasting at 8 pm on Saturday, you consume nothing except liquids until 8 pm on Sunday. Twenty-four hours fast is a natural way to detox the body that gives the digestive system a much-needed rest. A 24-hour fast is easy to incorporate into your everyday life. Just skip breakfast in the morning and sleep a little longer. You save time on grocery shopping and you save money. And at the end of the day, make it home and have your dinner. That's all, you will have done your full-day fast before you realize it.

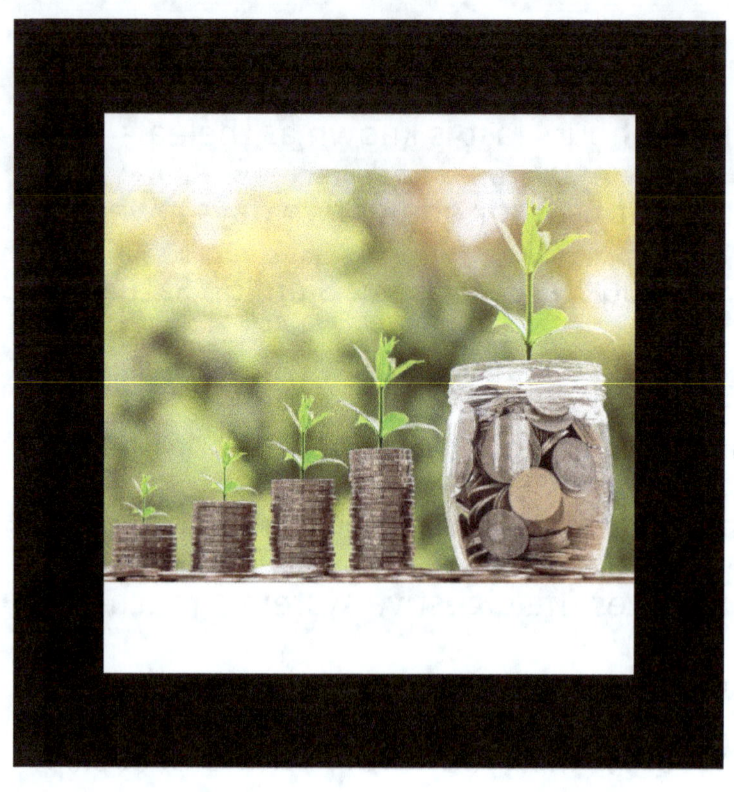

Save Time

Save Money

Lose Weight

Increase Health

The bottom line:

It's perfectly okay to try each of these methods before settling on the one that works best for you. All new things bring new challenges, just know that the body does gradually adapt to going without food or drastically limiting food intake as in the 5:2 diet. Keep yourself motivated by keeping your health goals top of mind, as well as the awesome benefits you will gain from fasting. Remember, you are doing it because you care about your health. Try to see it as a new challenge and an exciting adventure you've never tried before. It can actually become a very positive and enjoyable experience!

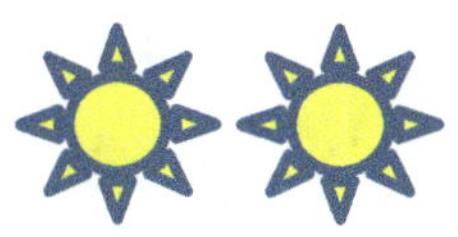

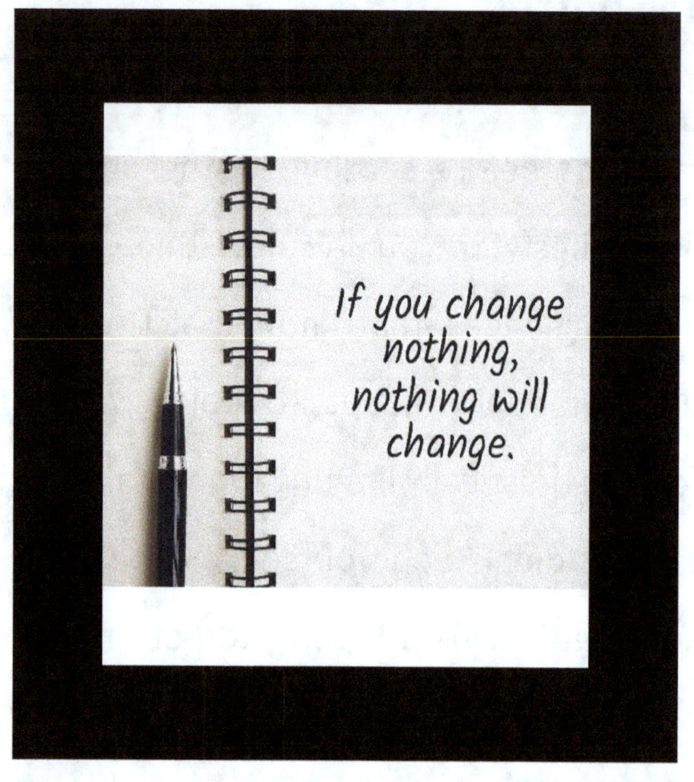

YOU ARE THE CREATOR

Possible Side Effects

Fasting can sometimes bring side effects, at least in the beginning. Being prepared for these will help you stay strong and conquer. The side effects are not life-threatening, therefore don't panic if you experience some of the following symptoms:

- Headache
- Drowsiness
- Irritability
- Mood swings
- Brain fog
- Fatigue
- A tendency to overeat and feel bloated
- Constipation
- Obsessing about food
- Hunger pains

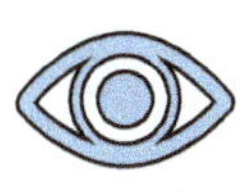
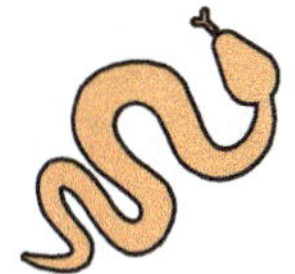

TRUST YOUR BODY

It is a natural reaction from the body to have these side effects as its course is changing from what it is used to. This will subside within a few days' time as your body gradually adapts itself to your new eating method.

However, if it doesn't reduce within 1-2 weeks' time, then this type of fasting is not the right course for you to take.

In some cases, intermittent fasting can cause hair loss, sleep disturbances and migraines. Although there is no severe risk involved even with these symptoms, it could be that, again, fasting is just not your thing.

STEP 3: Start Simple

Another way to prepare yourself physically and mentally is to start with small steps. Rather than choosing an intermittent fasting plan and jumping into it right away, try the following for a week or two until you feel more comfortable with depriving yourself of food.

- **Skip breakfast.**

Have some unsweetened herbal tea or coffee in the morning and don't eat anything else until lunchtime. Do this for one week. It's a great way to ease into the real thing.

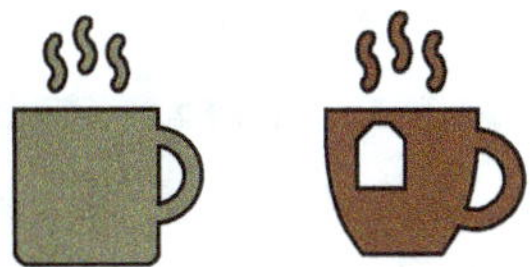

- **Don't snack.** Intermittent fasting can be particularly challenging if you are used to grazing or snacking through ought the day. Prepare yourself by cutting out all snacks between meals for a whole week before starting your fasting plan.

- **Don't eat after dinner.** Make dinner your absolute final meal of the day. Eat nothing and drink nothing except water until breakfast the next day.

> "Intermittent fasting can be a mental challenge as well as a physical one."

EMPOWER YOURSELF

However, it doesn't take long to overcome these hurdles once you get the hang of it. The side effects will gradually disappear, your body will adapt and you will begin to notice the amazing impact that fasting will have on your health. That will be all the motivation you need to keep going!

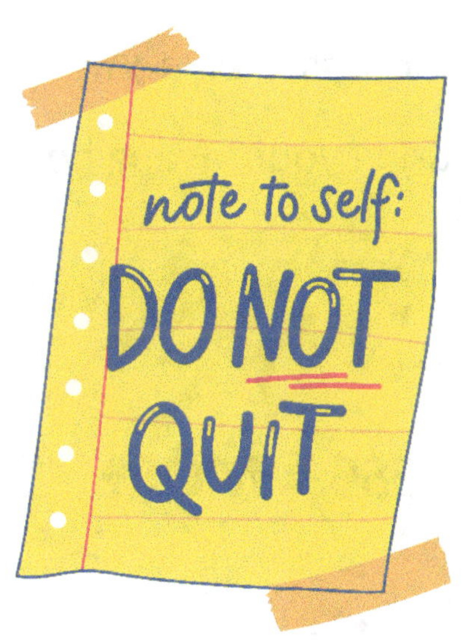

STEP 4:

Nutrition – Making Every Meal Count

Whatever your fasting plan, bear in mind that ultimately, you will be eating less. So, applying the "less is more" philosophy is the best way to make fasting work for you. That simply means making the most of what you eat by planning nutrition-packed meals that help you stay more full, more energized and less likely to miss essential nutrients during your fasting hours.

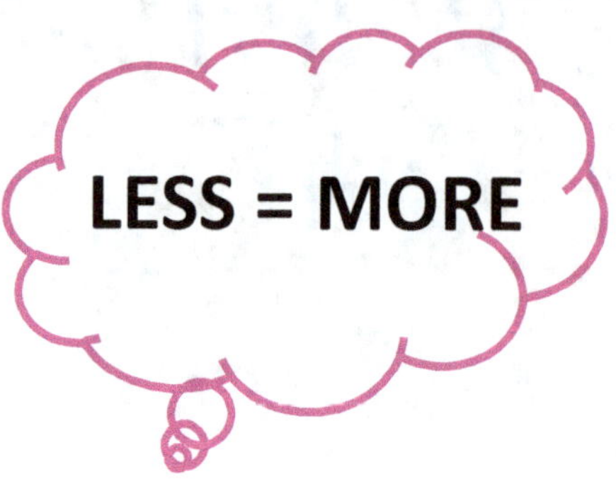

Being Hungry makes you stronger

Modern science say's that, 'what doesn't kill you makes you stronger. I.F. helps to recognize the difference between emotional eating and real hunger. Food is everywhere available to us that most of the time we are in the fed state. Most people don't experience real hunger. Then why is it that when we wake up in the morning, within an hour we start to feel hungry? Because your body is still digesting the food from your previous meal. And what you are experiencing is a habitual reaction to eat. You are simply eating out of habit, and in most cases, it is emotional eating.

ADDICTION

Besides eating being a habit, of course, your hormones are to be blamed as they adapt to whatever eating pattern you follow.

So, we don't just eat because we are hungry, we eat because we think we need to because we are addicted to sugar and fried foods. We get addicted to sugar and fried foods because they release **opioids and dopamine** in our bodies, just like addictive drugs do.

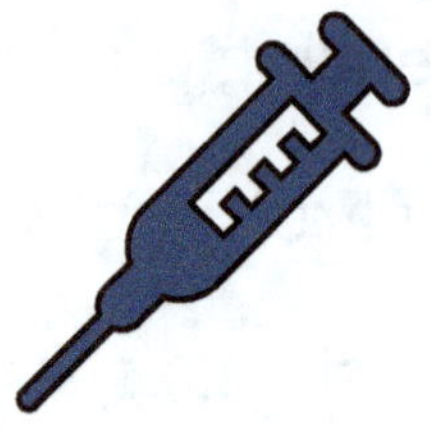

Hormones

The human growth hormone is produced by our brain's pituitary gland that stimulates growth, cell reproduction, and cell repair. It is thus crucial in human development and it pays an important role in slowing down the aging process. Intermittent fasting helps improve insulin sensitivity and increase human growth hormone. Let's talk about how intermittent fasting can help improve your hormonal profile.

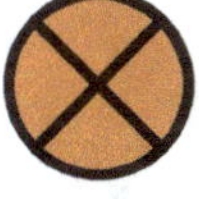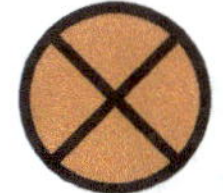

INSULIN

We start with insulin. Insulin is a hormone that it is released by the beta cells of your pancreas. Insulin helps sugar move from your blood to your cells, where it is used for energy. If you eat too many carbs in the form of processed sugar, like sweets and cakes, more insulin is released and the body needs to combat that extra sugar. Over time, your cells become in-sensitive to the excess insulin, leading to insulin sensitivity.

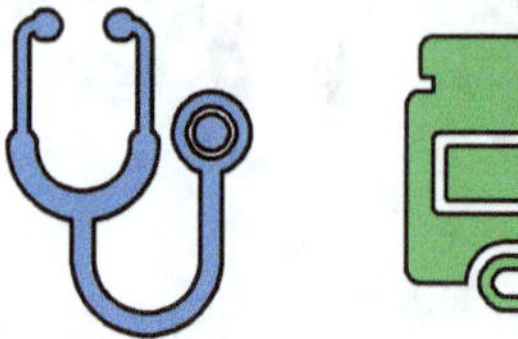

Fasting improves insulin sensitivity

A person with a high insulin level has a significantly increased risk of developing cardiovascular disease and diabetes. Scientific studies show that Intermittent fasting can lead to improved insulin sensitivity and reduces diabetes and heart disease.

Source: Healthline/Reduce Diabetes

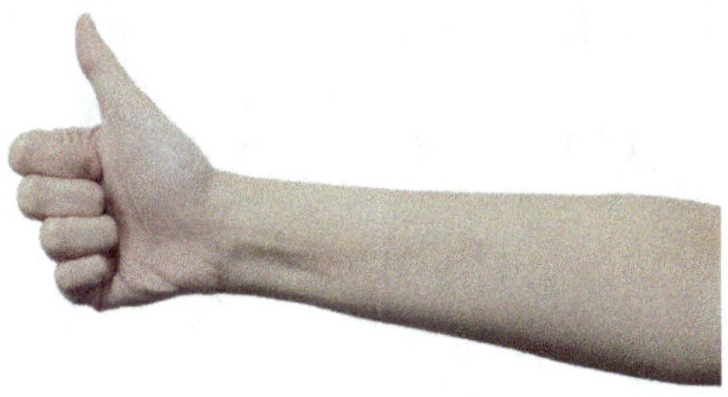

CHAPTER 4: What to Eat

Organic: Try to eat unprocessed organic food, with the right food you have more power, you keep looking good, and you'll last longer. The advantage of organic food is that it has a higher vibration fre-quency. It 'lives, like fruits and vegeta-bles, which means that the food contains more light particles. Our cells can absorb this strong light frequency, which allows them to swing back and forth at a higher speed. The high speed gives a higher state of regularity and an improvement in the functioning of your cells.

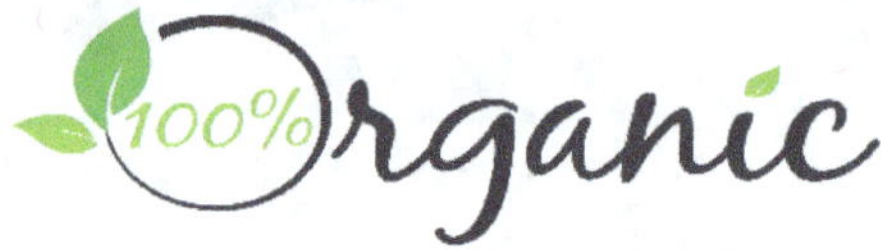

FIBERS

Maybe organic food is a little more expensive, but as you are eating fewer meals you save money and this you can put into organically-raised food including eggs, poultry, grass-fed beef, lamb and fish. • **Fibers:** Have an important role. They bring various benefits that are essential for the healthy digestive system of your body. *It regulates the body's use of sugars, helping to keep hunger and blood sugar in check.* Your digestive system loves eating foods high in fiber that are found in fresh green vegetables and fruits. Fiber also helps regulate your bowel movements and guards against constipation.

CARBS

 When you decide to eat healthier, you want to break up with as many unhealthy foods as you can. One of the first to go is usually carbs. Consuming too few calories or carbs can cause imbalances that can have severe consequences, including im-paired fertility, low mood, and weight gain. The good thing is that not all carbs mess with your health: Healthy carbs such as whole wheat grains, vegetables, whole-wheat pasta, wild rice, potatoes and yams will not only keep you fuller, they boost your energy levels and diges-tion.

Healthy Fats

Your body needs healthy fats that are primarily found in fish, olive oil and grass-fed butter. Fat is a source of essential fatty acids that the body cannot make. So why is fat a necessary part of a healthy, balanced diet? *Fat is a conductor that helps the body absorb vitamin A, vitamin D, and vitamin E.*

These vitamins are fat-soluble, which means they can only be absorbed with the help of fats.

Reminder

Remember that Intermittent fasting is simply one of many lifestyle strategies to improve your health, burn maximal fat, and help your body utilize the protein better so it can build more muscle without any food restrictions. Don't be too strict and wear yourself out over minute details. Try to eat your favorite foods in moderation; make sure to balance them out with many greens, fresh fruits and other healthy foods.

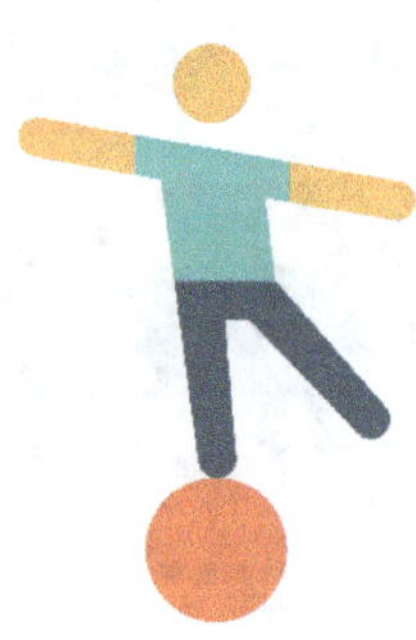

Taste Buds Improvement

The good thing about fasting is that it improves the sensitivity of your taste buds. Even your least favorite foods will seem appetizing when you're hungry—a terrific opportunity for you to adopt healthier and lasting eating habits by focusing on nutritious options. After a while, even a bowl of raw spinach can become the most delicious dish when you are fasting.

So, let your hunger help you eat healthier and introduce nutritious, healthy foods into your meals. Source: Nature.com

Giving up too fast

We live in a day in age where we want everything instantly. However, YouTube and social media indicate that you can fulfil any wish immediately; this distorts expectations. We want fast results, including health benefits and weight loss. But intermittent fasting is not a quick fix when it comes to weight loss or optimal health. It's an ancient practice that can get you excellent results, but only if practiced diligently long enough.

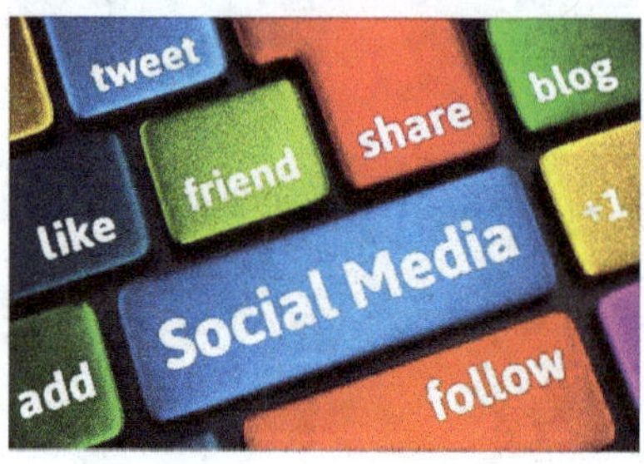

STEP 5: Organize high/low activity

There are many pros to intermittent fasting, and one of them is that you can easily accommodate it into your lifestyle and schedule. The key is to plan your fasting on days that are less active. Here are some tips on sailing through those fasting days more smoothly. **Schedule 24-hour fasts on weekends.** Believe me, extended fasts are never easy. I know because I have done it many times. What works best for me is to schedule a 24- hour fast on weekends when you have all the time to relax and spend time enjoying the activities you like or to take a long nap so that you conserve more energy.

Exercise on non-fasting days. If you are an athlete or simply work out regularly, always schedule these intensive exercise days when you are not fasting.

Accommodate your work schedule to your fasting. If you're lucky enough to do this, you will have a more enjoyable fasting experience. If possible, schedule important meetings and tasks that require more focus and concentration for days when you are not fasting. Again, if you work shifts, try to schedule your fasting around them. If you're eating window falls when you are at work, do try to bring a healthy pre-prepared meal from home rather than ordering fast food.

Motivating or de-motivating

I know that despite your planning, there will be those inevitable stressful, chaotic days that will come around while you are fasting. An important factor is how you speak with yourself. Are you motivating or de-motivating? Trust yourself and your body, it is a fantastic machine, a healthy person can survive a long period without eating because the blood sugar level regulates itself automatically. You can read about this in a scientific study from the National Library of Medicine, where blood sugar was not affected even after 84 hours of fasting. Source: PubMed

BE MINDFUL

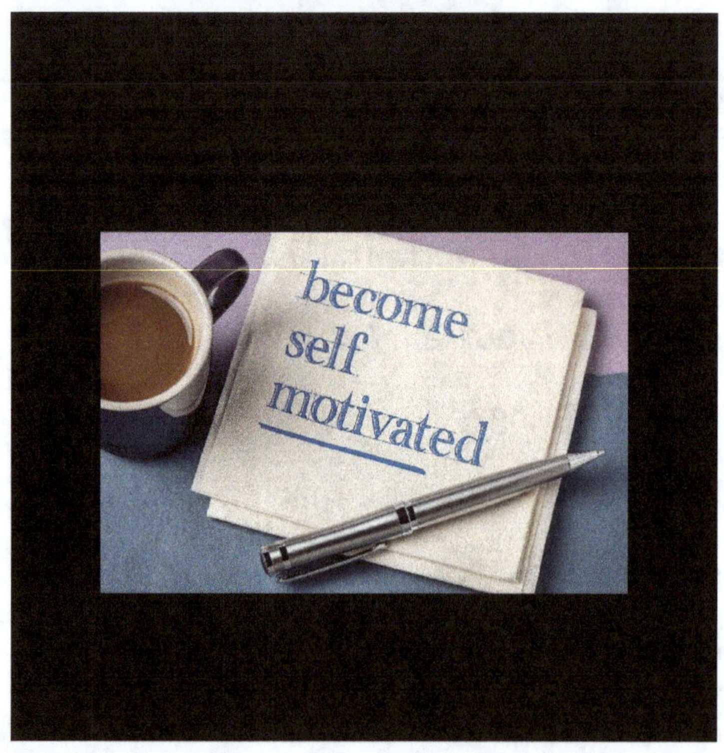

It is your Superpower

CHAPTER 5: Helpful Tips

Let your instincts guide you and consider these little tips and tweaks as you get into your fasting routine. Most of them are just plain common sense, but it's helpful to keep them in mind.

1. Stay hydrated. I recommend drinking plenty of water while you're fasting to avoid dehydration. The U.S. National Academies of Sciences, Engineering, and Medicine determined that an adequate daily fluid intake is: About 15.5 cups (3.7 liters) of fluids a day for men. About 11.5 cups (2.7 liters) of fluids a day for women.

Water also dulls hunger

So, that's a bonus. Try 1–2 teaspoons apple cider vinegar per day mixed in a large glass of water. Japanese scientists found that drinking vinegar might help fight obesity, but taking too much can cause problems, like eroding the enamel of your teeth. Unsweetened herbal tea, hot or cold, is another excellent alternative or coffee to perk you up in the morning may enhance the benefits of intermittent fasting, including reduced inflammation and improved brain function. If you don't like to drink it black, add a few drops of milk or cream.

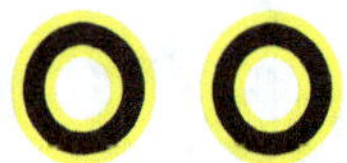

2. Consume whole, healthy foods.

Do you need vitamin supplements with I.F? When you eat whole, healthy foods like fruit, vegetables, protein, and healthy grains, it's unlikely you'll become deficient in crucial vitamins and minerals. But every person is different. If you feel like something is off, consult your general practitioner. If you feel great, you can continue the course. I.F does have the potential to trigger hormonal reactions, especially when you take it to the extreme and it causes you to feel stressed. Remember that Intermittent Fasting is a means to be mindful and enjoy a healthy body, and Stress is detrimental to your physical and mental health.

3. Get into the sun. Sunlight helps your body produce vitamin D. Vitamin D is important because it regulates the body's day and night rhythm and it will help your body cycle adapt to fasting much faster. Therefore, go outside as much as you can.

4. Don't force yourself. Stay Honest with yourself, this is the best policy when it comes to intermittent fasting. If you simply can't function normally and the hunger and discomfort are just too extreme, it's time to call it quits. It doesn't mean you're weak or that you lack willpower, it only means that,

Intermittent fasting is not your thing.

5. Eat slowly when you break your fast.

In the first few days of your fast, when your body is learning to adjust to the new program, you can feel so hungry that you end up eating too fast, leaving you feeling bloated and uncomfortable. When you sit down to eat, be mindful and take small mouthfuls. While slowly eating increases your enjoyment of food, it can also improve digestion.

6. Don't overeat. After your fasting period, you will have an extended eating window; you can continue to eat during this time but try not to eat it all at once!

Consider having a light and nutritious meal and stop eating when your hunger is moderately satisfied. It's not good to overfill your stomach because it will go into overdrive after being without food for so long. Overeating will leave you feeling bloated and very uncomfortable.

7. Experiment with different fasting times. Choosing to experiment with different available approaches of I.F can help you discover a strategy that best works for you. Assess your lifestyle, work and commitments to find the best times for you.

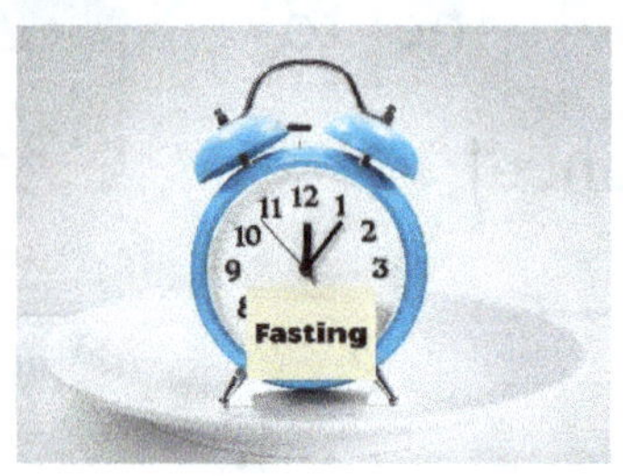

Last year, for example, I was flying abroad to visit friends, and I didn't eat that day. Due to the flight delay and skipping the poor nutrition on the plane, it ended up being 26 hours between meals. For me, this was the longest time without eating.

8. Commitment. I have a hectic agenda, and I want to keep my mind as straightforward as possible. To combine these together requires two things, one, commitment and two, a simple fasting app that help me stay on track.

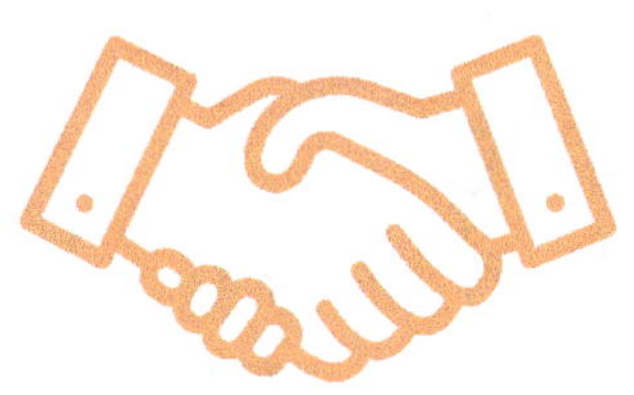

9. A fasting app. can do everything from organizing your fasting schedule, alerting you to mealtimes, helping you plan meals and even tracking your weight. There's a great variety of fasting apps available online for free, and they are super easy to use.

10. Journal your progress. Keeping a journal can be a great idea to keep you motivated and excited about the changes you will experience. You can use it to record your feelings every few days, as well as weight loss and other improvements you start to notice.

Conclusion

Now you have all the basics you need to start your intermittent fasting routine, and within a few days, you will begin to see and feel the powerful benefits of intermittent fasting. Your belly will begin to disappear as you lose weight. You gain more energy and mental clarity, your digestion improves, and you will feel so much healthier. Enjoy yourself knowing that Your mindset is what creates the line between success and failure.

With a positive and excited mindset, intermittent fasting can become an enjoyable experience.

Follow the simple steps and tips provided here to help you quick- start and then ease into a successful – and hopefully, a consistent – fasting routine.

Then, do more research if you need to, and consult your doctor if you have any further doubts.

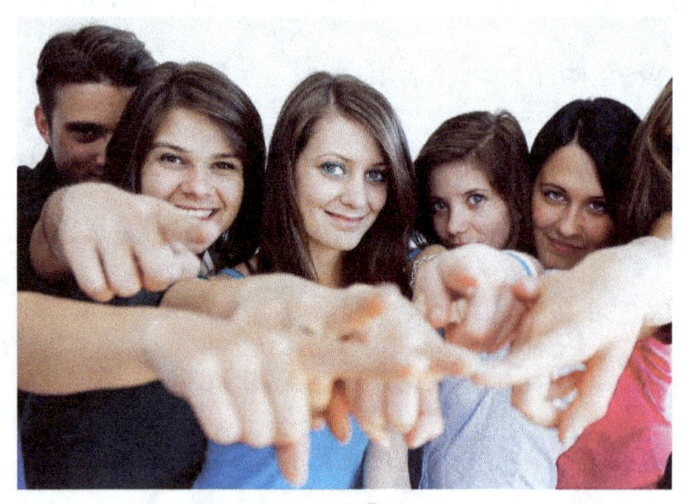

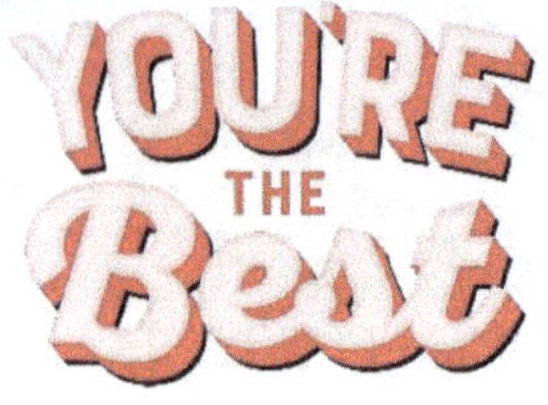

And finally

I love Intermittent Fasting, and I am sure I will do it for the rest of my life. Not only for the superior health benefits and peace of mind, but it saves me a LOT of time as well. Own it, so don't overthink; embrace it with an open mind and see where it takes you.

Enjoy Your New Intermittent Fasting Life-style!

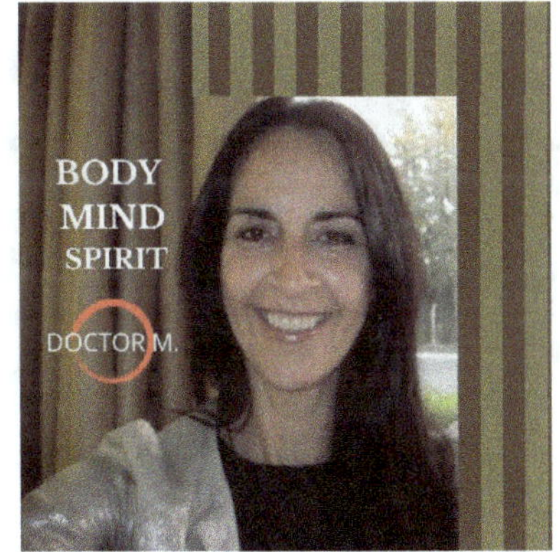

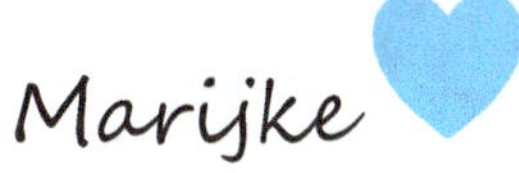

Marijke

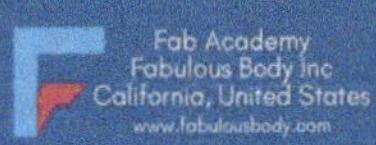

DIPLOMA
IN INTERMITTENT FASTING

This Certificate is Proudly Presented to

Dr. Marijke Verkerk

Grade: Distinction

Has successfully completed this Internationally Accredited CPD Activity

May you Inspire Others with your exemplary performance

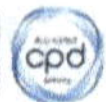

16 August 2020

DATE

AUTHORIZED SIGNATORY

BODY | MIND | SPIRIT

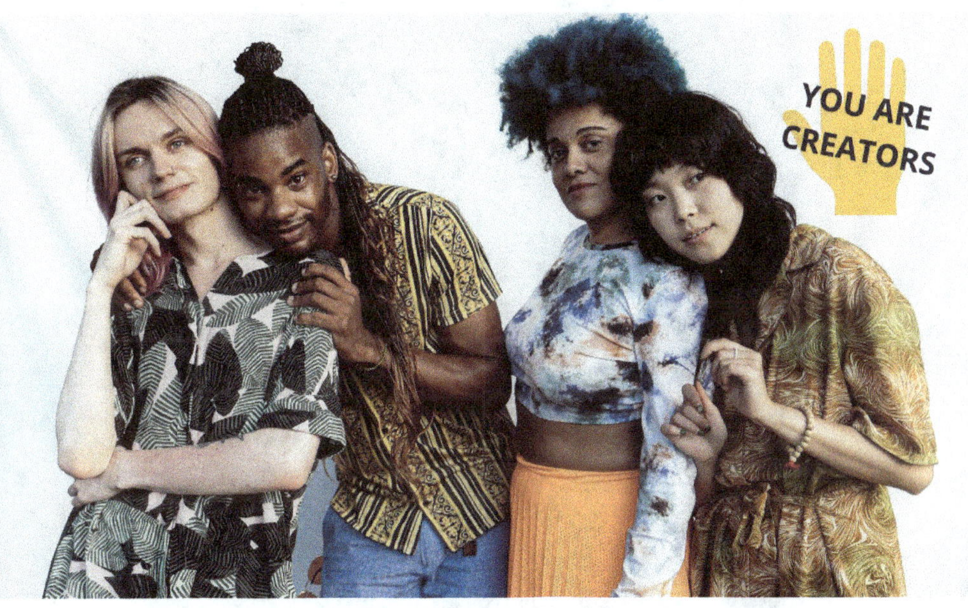

I started Body | Mind | Spirit with a simple vision: to create a place that you can visit when you're looking for inspiration or motivation and gain instant clarity on who you are and what kind of life you want to be living.

MASTER CREATORS WITH A SINGLE MISSION

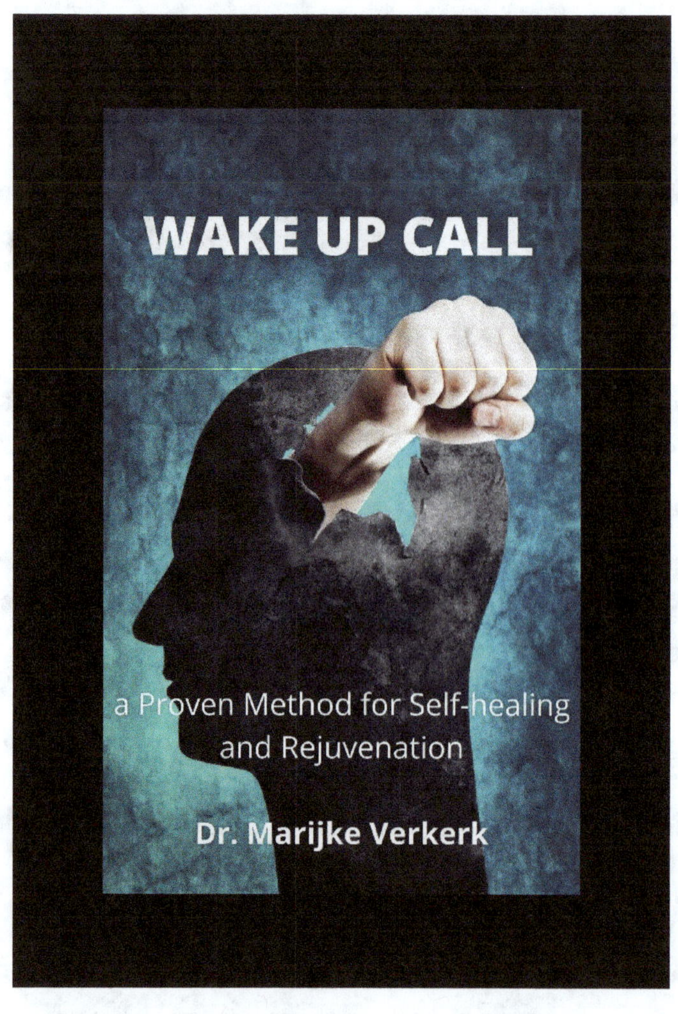

Wake Up Call

a Proven Method for Self-healing
and Rejuvenation
Dr. Marijke Verkerk